Preface

The standardized Scalp Acupuncture Manipulation was drawn up by the World Federation of Acupuncture – Moxibustion Societies. Annex A of this standard is informative. Annex B of this standard is normative.

Supporting institutions: Changchun University of Traditional Chinese Medicine, Changchun, China.

Mainauthors: Wang Fuchun.

Assistant authors: Jiao Shunfa, Yan Xingke, Wang Hongfeng, Li Tie, Gao Ying, Zhou Dan, Xu Xiaohong, Gao Shuzhong.

International Members of the working group: Ken Lubowich (America), Liu Shuquan (Australia), Liu Tieying (England), Yu Qunling (Canada), Wang Fuchun (China), Jiao Shunfa (China), Lee Junmo (Korea), Megumi Masumoto (Japan), Liu Jiqiu (Singapore), Xia Linjun (Hungary).

International Observers: Kurihara Wan Lizi (Japan), Wang Bangkun (Singapore).

U0346166

1 Scope

The standard defines the terms, definitions, operation steps, requirements, operation methods, attentions and taboos of scalp acupuncture.

The standard applies to the use of the manipulations of scalp acupuncture.

2 Terms and Definitions

For the purposes of this document, the following terms and definitions apply.

2.1 Scalp Acupuncture

Scalp acupuncture is a therapeutic method to puncture specific point – line on the scalp with needles.

2.2 Subcutaneous Needling

The needle is inserted subcutaneously with an angle of about $15° \sim 30°$ between the needle shaft and the scalp. The method is also known as transverse insertion.

3 Operation Steps and Requirements

3.1 Preparation

3.1.1 Needles

Filiform needles should be selected according to patients' conditions and scalp site. The needles must have polished and straight bodies (shafts) without rusts or bends, solid handle and sharp tips without barbs.

3.1.2 Locations

Select locations according to different disease. The locations and indications of scalp acupuncture are presented in Annex A.

3.1.3 Patient' Body Position for Treatment

The sitting position is appropriate, or selects a position comfortable for patient and convenient for practitioner.

3.1.4 Environmental Setting for Treatment

Be sure that the environment setting should be clean and no pollutant.

3.1.5 Sterilization

3.1.5.1 Sterilization of Needles

It is better to select the disposable filiform needles. Reusable needles should be processed with high – pressure sterilization method according to international inspection standards (ISO 11737).

3.1.5.2 Disinfection of the Skin Selected for Acupuncture

The location should be disinfected with 75% alcohol cotton or 1% iodophor ball in a circular motion from the center to the periphery, according to international inspection standards (ISO 11737).

3.1.5.3 Personal Hygiene of the Acupuncturists

Before operation the acupuncturist should wash hands with soapsuds, then disinfect with 75% alcohol cotton ball according tointernational inspection standards (ISO 11737).

3.2 Needling Methods

3.2.1 Angle of Insertion

Normally the needles are inserted obliquely with an angle of about $15° \sim 30°$ between the needle shaft and the skin, then the needle is inserted horizontally into the skin.

3.2.2 Fast Insertion

Insert the needle into the subgaleal region rapidly and parallel to the skin to reach certain depth.

3.2.3 Depth of Insertion

After the needle is inserted into the layer beneath the galea aponeurotica, the needle should be inserted along the skin; the depth of insertion depends on the patient's condition and the requirements of the prescription.

3. 2. 4   Needle Manipulation

After the needle body enters the layer beneath the galea aponeurotic, the acupuncturist should immobilize the shoulder, elbow, and wrist joints and thumb to prevent the needle from moving. Bend the proximal and distal joints of index finger as semi – buckling state, and hold the needle handle with the palm side of the thumb and the radial surface of the index finger. Twist the needle by bending and stretching movement of the metacarpophalangeal joint of the index finger rapidly without stopping, at a frequency of 200 times per minute, and last for at least 1 ~ 3 minutes.

During the process of treatment, the needles are manipulated intermittently. To strengthen the stimulation and achieve better effect repetitively twirl the needles for about 2 ~ 3 times. Each twirling may last 1 ~ 3 minutes.

3. 2. 5   Needle Retention

In general needles are retained for 15 ~ 30 minutes, but retention for 2 ~ 24 hours may be used for severe or complicated cases. Prescribe the patients to do exercises during needle retention can enhance the therapeutic effect. Manipulation is not needed during the needle retention.

3. 2. 6   Withdrawal of the Needle

Withdraw the needle quickly and press the puncture hole with a dry sterilized cotton ball for a while to prevent bleeding.

3. 2. 7   Management of Possible Accidents

Annex B presents methods of management for fainting, stuck needle, bent needle, broken needle or hematoma during or after treatment.

4   Precautions

4. 1   A small part the needle shaft should be exposed outside the scalp during the needle retention. Do not disturb the needles under the skin to avoid bending or breaking. If the patient feels discomfort in needling site, withdraw the needle 0. 1 ~ 0. 2cm. Special attentions should be paid to patients with severe cardio – cerebrovascular diseases during the period of needle retention.

4. 2   Be cautious when treating the patients who are nervous, hungry, or overeat. Strong manipulation is not advised.

4. 3   Carefully check the number of the needles after the needle withdrawal in order to ensure no needles are left.

5   Contraindication

Scalp acupuncture should not be used in the following cases.

5. 1   Infants whose fontanel and seams of the skull are not closed.

5. 2   Patients who have skull defects, open brain injury, severe inflammation, ulcers or scars.

5. 3   Patients who are suffering from severe heart disease, diabetes, anemia, acute inflammation or cardiac failure.

5. 4   Patients who are suffering from stroke should be treated only after their blood pressure and disease conditions were stable.

Annex A

(Informative)

International Standard Proposal of Scalp Acupuncture Point Line

A. 1   International Standard Proposal of Scalp Acupuncture Point Line

A. 1. 1 MS_1 Ezhongxian (Middle Line of Forehead)

Midle mid – sagittal line of forehead, 1 cun long from Shenting (DU_{24}) straight downward, extending 0. 5 cun superior and inferior anterior to the hairline, belongs to the Governor Vessel.

A. 1. 2 MS_2 Epangxian I (Lateral Line 1 of Forehead)

Line 1 lateral to mid – sagittal line, superior to the inner canthus, 1 cun long from Meichong (BL_3) straight downward, belongs to the Bladder Meridian.

A. 1. 3 MS_3 Epangxian ‖ (Lateral Line 2 of Forehead)

Line 2 lateral to forehead, 1 cun long from Toulinqi (GB_{15}) straight downward, superior to the pupil, belongs to Gall Bladder Meridian.

A. 1. 4 MS_4 Epangxian ‖‖ (Lateral Line 3 of Forehead)

Line 3 lateral to forehead, 1 cun long, 0. 75 cun medial to Touwei (ST_8) straight downward, 0. 5 cun superior and inferior to the hairline, between Gall Bladder and Bladder Meridians.

A. 1. 5 MS_5 Dingzhongxian (Middle Line of Vertex)

Middle line of vertex, extending from Baihui (DU_{20}) interiorly to Qianding (DU_{21}), belongs to Governor Vessel.

A. 1. 6 MS_6 Dingnie Qianxiexian (Anterior Oblique Line of Vertex – Temporal)

From Qian Sishencong ($EX – HN_1$) oblique to Xuanli(GB_6). It traverses the Gall Bladder and Bladder Meridians diagonally.

A. 1. 7 MS_7 Dingnie Houxiexian (Posterior Oblique Line of Vertex – Temporal)

From Baihui (DU_{20}) obliquely to Qubin (GB_7). It traverses the Governor Vessel, Gall Bladder and Bladder Meridians diagonally.

A. 1. 8 MS_8 Dingpangxian I (Line 1 Lateral to Vertex)

Bilaterally 1. 5 cun lateral to middle line of vertex, 1. 5 cun long posteriorly from Chengguang (BL_6) belongs to the Bladder Meridian.

A. 1. 9 MS_9 Dingpangxian ‖ (Line 2 Lateral to Vertex)

Bilaterally 2. 25 cun 1 ateral to middle line of vertex, 1. 5 cun posteriorly from Zhengying (GB_{17}) belongs to the Gall Bladder Meridian.

A. 1. 10 MS_{10} Nieqianxian (Anterior Temporal Line)

From Hanyan(GB_4) to XuanLi (GB_6), belongs to Gall Bladder Meridian.

A. 1. 11 MS_{11} Niehouxian (Posterior Temporal Line)

From Shuaigu (GB_8) to Qubin (GB_7), belongs to Gall Bladder Meridian.

A. 1. 12 MS_{12} Zhenshang Zhengzhong xian (Upper – Middle Line of Occiput)

From Qiangjian (DU_{18}) to Naohu (DU_{17}), belongs to Governor Vessel.

A. 1. 13 MS$_{13}$ Zhenshang Pangxian (Upper – Middle Line of Occiput)

0. 5 cun lateral and parallel to upper – middle line of occiput.

A. 1. 14 MS$_{14}$ Zhenxia Pangxian (Lower – Lateral Line of Occiput)

2 cun long from Yuzhen (BL$_9$) straightly inferior, belongs to Bladder Meridian.

A. 2 Location and Indications

A. 2. 1 Forehead Area (Chart A1)

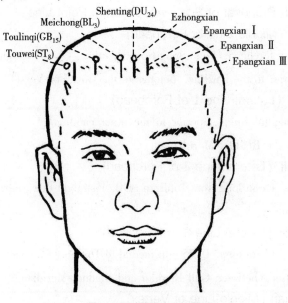

Chart A1 Anterior View

A. 2. 1. 1 Middle Line of Forehead MS$_1$ Ezhongxian

Location: This line is in the middle of the forehead, running 0. 5 cun superiorly and inferiorly respectively to the anterior hair line. Acupuncture needle is inserted into DU$_{24}$ (Shenting), reaching 1 cun anterio – inferiorly. It is on the Governor Vessel.

Indications: Headache, involuntary laughing, weeping, insomnia, amnesia, dream – disturbed sleep, mania and nasal disorders.

A. 2. 1. 2 Lateral Line of Forehead MS$_2$ Epangxian Ⅰ

Location: This line is lateral to the middle line of forehead, and on the line linking the inner canthus. It extends between 0. 5 cun superior and inferior to the hair line. Acupuncture needle is inserted into to BL$_3$ (Meichong), reaching 1 cun anterio – inferiorly. It is on the Bladder Meridian.

Indications: Disorders of the upper – jiao, such as coronary heart disease, angina pectoris, bronchial asthma, bronchitis and insomnia.

A. 2. 1. 3 Lateral Line 2 of Forehead MS$_3$ Epangxian Ⅱ

Location: This line is lateral to MS$_2$, and superior to the pupils, extending 0. 5 cun superior and inferior to the hair line. Acupuncture needle is inserted into GB$_{15}$ (Toulinqi), reaching 1 cun anterio – inferiorly. It is on the Gallbladder Meridian.

Indications: Disorders of the middle – jiao, such as acute or chronic gastritis, gastro – duodenal ulcer and liver – gallbladder diseases.

A. 2. 1. 4 Lateral Line 3 of Forehead MS$_4$ Epangxian Ⅲ

Location: This line is lateral to MS$_3$. Acupuncture needle is applied to the place 0. 75 cun medial to ST$_8$

(Touwei), a line extending 0.5 cun superior and inferior the hair line. It is the midline between the Gallbladder and Stomach Meridians.

Indications: Disorders of the lower – jiao, such as functional uterine bleeding, impotence, seminal emission, uterine prolapse, above and below frequent and urgent urination.

A.2.2 Vertex Area (Chart A2 ~ A3)

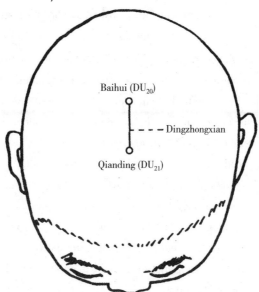

Chart A2   Top of Head

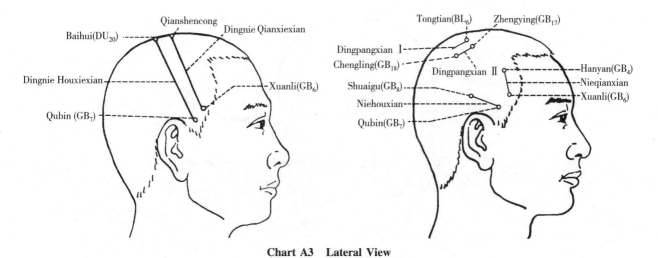

Chart A3   Lateral View

A.2.2.1 Middle Line of Vertex MS$_5$ Dingzhongxian

Location: This line is on the mid – sagittal line of vertex. Acupuncture needle is applied to the line 1.5 cun from DU$_{20}$(Baihui) to DU$_{21}$(Qianding). It is on the Governor Vessel.

Indications: Disorders of lower back, leg and foot, such as paralysis, numbness, pain, cortical polyuria, nocturia in children, prolapse of rectum, gastroptosis, prolapse of uterus, high blood pressure and pain in the top of head.

A.2.2.2 Anterior Oblique Line of Vertex – Temporal MS$_6$ Dingnieqianxiexian

Location: This line is on the temporal side of the head, on the line linking EX – HN$_1$ (Qian Sishencong) and GB₆(Xuanli), which obliquely passes through the Bladder and Gallbladder Meridians.

Indications: It is effective for central motor dysfunction of the contralateral limbs. The line is divided into 5 equal segments. Acupuncture applied to the upper 1/5, the middle and lower 2/5, and is used for contralateral central paralysis of the lower limbs, contralateral central paralysis of the upper limbs and facial, motor aphasia, salivation and cerebral arteriosclerosis respectively.

A. 2. 2. 3   Posterior Oblique Line of Vertex – Temporal MS₇ Dingniehouxiexian

Location: This line is on the temporal side of the head, on the line linking DU₂₀(Baihui) and GB₇(Qubin), and it obliquely passes through the Governor Vessel, Bladder and Gallbladder Meridians.

Indications: It is effective for central sensory disturbance of contralateral limbs. The line is divided into 5 equal segments. Acupuncture needle is applied to the upper 1/5, the middle and lower 2/5, for contralateral sensory disturbance of the lower limbs, the upper limbs, the head and face, respectively.

A. 2. 2. 4   Lateral Line 1 of Vertex MS₈ Dingpangxian I

Location: This is on the top of the head, 1. 5 cun lateral to and parallel to the middle line of vertex. Acupuncture needle is applied to BL₆(Chengguang) posteriorly reaching 1. 5 cun. It is on the Bladder Meridian.

Indications: Disorders of the lower back, leg and foot, such as paralysis, numbness and pain.

A. 2. 2. 5   Lateral Line 2 of Vertex MS₉ Dingpangxian II

Location: This line is on the top of the head, 0. 75 cun laterals to the lateral line 1 of vertex and 2. 25 cun laterals to the middle line of vertex. Acupuncture needle is applied to GB₁₇(Zhengying) posteriorly reaching 1. 5 cun. It is on the Gallbladder Meridian.

Indication: Disorders of the shoulder, arm and hand, such as paralysis, numbness and pain.

A. 2. 3   Temporal Area (Chart A4)

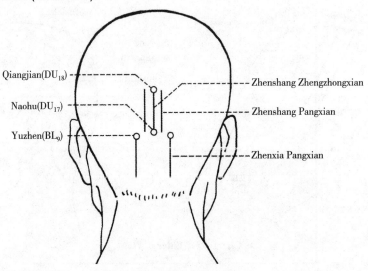

Chart A4   Posterior View

A. 2. 3. 1   Anterior Temporal Line MS₁₀ Nieqianxian

Location: This line is on the temporal side of the head, on the line linking GB₄(Hanyan) and GB₆(Xuanli). It is on the Gallbladder Meridian.

Indications: Migraine, motor aphasia, peripheral facial palsy and oral disease.

A. 2. 3. 2   Posterior Temporal Line MS₁₁ Niehouxian

Location: This line is on the temporal side of the head, directly above the ear apex, on the line linking

GB$_8$(Shuaigu) and GB$_7$(Qubin). It is on the Gallbladder Meridian.

Indications: Migraine, dizziness, deafness and tinnitus.

A. 2. 4   Occipital Area

A. 2. 4. 1   Upper Middle Line of Occiput MS$_{12}$ Zhenshangzhengzhongxian

Location: This line is on the occipital area, on the mid – sagittal line superior to the external occipital protuberance, on the line linking DU$_{18}$(Qiangjian) and DU$_{17}$(Naohu). It is on the Governor Vessel.

Indications: Eye diseases.

A. 2. 4. 2   Upper Lateral Line of Occiput MS$_{13}$ Zhenshangpangxian

Location: This line is on the occipital area, on the line 0. 5 cun lateral to and parallel to the upper middle line of occiput.

Indications: Eye diseases, such as cortical visual disorder, cataract, nearsightedness and painful conjunctivitis.

A. 2. 4. 3   Lower Lateral Line of Occiput MS$_{14}$ Zhenxiapangxian

Location: This line is on the occipital area. It is 2 cun long from BL$_9$(Yuzhen), extending inferiorly. It is on the Bladder Meridian.

Indications: Balance disturbance, posterior headache and bilateral pain of the lower back and imbalance due to cerebellum disease.

Annex B

(Normative)

Methods of Management for Fainting, Stuck Needle, Bent Needle, Broken Needle or Hematoma during or after Treatment

B. 1 Fainting during Acupuncture Treatment

B. 1. 1 Clinical Manifestation of Fainting

The symptoms of fainting during scalp acupuncture include listlessness, dizziness, blurred vision, pale face, nausea, vomiting, excessive sweating, palpitation, cold limbs, hypotension, weak and thready pulse, or coma, cyanosis of the lips and nails, urinary and fecal incontinence, and a small and thin pulse as if expiring.

B. 1. 2 Management

Stop manipulation and withdraw all the needles immediately. Arrange the patient to lie down and keep warm. The mild case can recover soon after lying down for a while and drinking plenty of hot water or sugared water. For severe case, in addition to the above measures, needle DU_{26}(Shuigou), PC_6(Neiguan), ST_{36}(Zusanli) or do moxibustion on DU_{20}(Baihui), RN_4(Guanyuan) and RN_6(Qihai). If a patient falls into a coma, necessary emergency care must be used immediately.

B. 1. 3 Precautions

B. 1. 3. 1 During the first visit, ask if the patient had previous acupuncture treatments fainting history due to the treatment. Then assess his physical constitution carefully and explain the scalp acupuncture treatment thoroughly. Do not offer treatment if the patient is unwilling to accept scalp acupuncture.

B. 1. 3. 2 If a patient has a history of fainting, should arrange a comfortable and safe position for treatment. Lying down is advised and selecting fewer points with mild stimulation. Use superficial needling without retaining the needles. When strong stimulation is needed, use an appropriate frequency, amplitude and intensity that patient can tolerate. Make patient gradually adjust to the treatment.

B. 1. 3. 3 Do not give scalp acupuncture to patients who are hungry, fatigued, or after overeating or drunkenness.

B. 1. 3. 4 During treatment closely observe the patient's expression and ask how he feels. In case of feeling discomfort proper procedures should be adopted immediately.

B. 2 Stuck Needling

B. 2. 1 Clinical Manifestations

Stuck needle is a common problem in scalp acupuncture. The doctor may experience a sticking feeling when twirling, lifting, thrusting or withdrawing the needle, meanwhile the patient feels pain.

B. 2. 2 Management

Prolong the duration of needle retention when a needle is stuck. Ask the patient to relax and use gentle massage around the needle.

B. 2. 3 Precautions

Stuck needle is often caused by rapid unidirectional twirling of a needle. Special attention should be paid to manipulation techniques. Manipulate the needle with even force and avoid unidirectional twirling.

B. 3   Bent or Broken Needle

B. 3. 1   Clinical Manifestations

The needle body (shaft) bends or breaks inside or outside the tissue.

B. 3. 2   Management

Stop lifting – thrusting or twirling when a needle is bent or broken. If needle body has slight bend, withdraw it gently. If the bend angle is over curved, withdraw it following the bending direction. Don't withdraw or rotate the needle forcefully to avoid breaking the needle in the patient's body. If the needle is broken, and its broken part protrudes from the skin, remove it with forceps. If the broken part is close to surface beneath the skin, compress the skin with fingers around the needle to expose the shaft, and then remove it with forceps. If the broken part is completely embedded under the skin, surgical removal is required under the X – ray.

B. 3. 3   Precautions

To prevent bending or breaking needles, it is necessary to check all needles carefully before using. Never use any rusted or bent needles. Also the patient should be told not to disturb the needle to prevent bends or breaks.

B. 4   Hematoma

B. 4. 1   Clinical Manifestations

Blood vessels are rich in scalp, tissues and needling may cause local pain when a inserting needles into scalp tissue or during needle retention. The needle hole may bleed after withdrawing the needle causing local swelling and pain.

B. 4. 2   Management

The micro subcutaneous hemorrhage does not need special care. It will disappear itself. If local swelling and pain is severe, alternatively apply cold and warm compresses to stop bleeding. Mild massage promotes the absorption of blood stasis and decrease the swelling.

B. 4. 3   Precautions

Before acupuncture treatment, examine needles carefully. Be familiar with the anatomy of head, and avoid puncturing the blood vessels. Press the needle hole with dry disinfected cotton balls after withdrawing the needle. Reduce the time for needle retention, withdraw the needle gently and fast in those who bleed easily, and press the needle hole immediately if bleeding.

前　言

头针技术操作规范由世界针灸学会联合会起草制定。本标准的附录 A 为资料性附录，附录 B 为规范性附录。

支持单位：长春中医药大学。

主要作者：王富春。

参与者：焦顺发、严兴科、王洪峰、李铁、高颖、周丹、徐晓红、高树中。

国际工作组成员：卢布威（美国）、刘树权（澳大利亚）、刘铁英（英格兰）、于群玲（加拿大）、王富春（中国）、焦顺发（中国）、李俊茂（韩国）、松本惠（日本）、刘冀秋（新加坡）、夏林军（匈牙利）。

国际观察员：栗原万里子（日本）、王邦坤（新加坡）。

1　范围

本标准规定了头针的术语与定义、操作步骤与要求、操作方法、注意事项、禁忌。

本标准适用于头针技术操作。

2　术语与定义

下列术语和定义适用于本标准。

2.1　头针

在头皮特定部位针刺的治疗方法，又称头皮针。

2.2　平刺法

进针时，针体和头皮穴线皮肤呈15°～30°角刺入的刺法，又称沿皮刺或横刺法。

3　操作步骤与要求

3.1　施术前准备

3.1.1　针具选择

针具选择：应根据病情和操作部位选择不同型号的毫针。应选择针身光滑、无锈蚀和折痕、针柄牢固、针尖锐利、无倒钩的针具。

3.1.2　穴线选择

穴线选择：应根据不同的疾病选用不同的头针穴线治疗。头针穴线定位、主治见附录A。

3.1.3　体位选择

体位选择：应选择患者舒适、医者便于操作的治疗体位。

3.1.4　环境要求

环境要求：应注意环境清洁卫生，避免污染。

3.1.5　消毒

3.1.5.1　针具消毒

应选择高压消毒法，宜选择一次性毫针。对于可重复使用的针具，应按照国际检查标准（ISO 11737），使用高压消毒法消毒。

3.1.5.2　部位消毒

根据国际检查标准（ISO 11737），施术之前，应选用75%医用乙醇或1%碘伏的棉球或棉签在施术部位由中心向外环擦拭。

3.1.5.3　术者消毒

根据国际检查标准（ISO 11737），施术之前，医者双手应用肥皂水清洗干净，再用75%医用乙醇消毒棉球擦拭。

3.2　施术方法

3.2.1　进针角度

一般宜在针体与皮肤呈15°～30°角进针，然后平刺进入穴线内。

3.2.2　快速进针

将针迅速刺入皮下，当针尖达到帽状腱膜下层时，指下感到阻力减小，然后使针与头皮平行，根据不同穴线刺入不同深度。

3.2.3　进针深度

一般情况下，针刺入帽状腱膜下层后，使针体平卧，进针深度宜根据患者的具体情况和处方要求决定。

3.2.4　行针

针体进入帽状腱膜下层后，术者肩、肘、腕关节和拇指固定不动，以保持毫针相对固定。食指第1、2节呈半屈曲状，用食指第1节的桡侧面与拇指第1节的掌侧面持住针柄，然后食指掌指关节做伸屈运动，使针体快速旋转，捻转频率以200次/分钟左右为宜，持续1~3分钟。

在整个治疗过程中，间歇操作捻针。为了加强刺激强度并保证良好的治疗效果，反复旋转针具2~3次，每次持续1~3分钟。

3.2.5 留针

留针期间不再施行任何针刺手法，让针体安静而自然地留置在头皮内。一般情况下，头针留针时间宜为15~30分钟。如症状严重、病情复杂、病程较长者，可留针2~24小时。留针期间，让患者辅以运动，可以加强治疗效果。此外，留针期间不需要再行操作。

3.2.6 出针

先缓慢出针至皮下，然后迅速拔出，拔针后必须用消毒干棉球按压针孔，以防出血。

3.2.7 施术异常情况的处理

头针施术过程中或施术后，如出现晕针、滞针、弯针、断针或血肿时，附录B给出了具体的处理方法。

4 注意事项

4.1 留针应注意安全，针体应稍露出头皮，不宜随意或盲目碰触留置在头皮下的毫针，以免折针、弯针。如在进针和留针中局部不适，可稍稍退出1~2分。对有严重心脑血管疾病而需要长期留针者，应加强监护，以免发生意外。

4.2 对体质虚弱或精神紧张、过饱或过饥者应慎用，不宜采取强刺激手法。

4.3 头发较密部位常易遗忘所刺入的毫针，起针时须反复检查，确保不会有针具遗漏。

5 禁忌

以下情况不宜接受头针治疗：

5.1 囟门和骨缝尚未骨化的婴儿。

5.2 头部颅骨缺损处或开放性脑损伤部位、所刺头皮有感染、溃疡、瘢痕者。

5.3 患有严重心脏病、重度糖尿病、重度贫血、急性炎症和心力衰竭者。

5.4 中风患者，急性期如因脑血管意外引起昏迷、血压过高时，暂不宜用头针治疗，须待血压和病情稳定后，方可做头针治疗。

附 录 A

（资料性附录）

头针穴名国际标准化方案

A. 1 头针穴名国际标准化方案

A. 1. 1 MS₁ Ezhongxian（额中线）

Middle line of forehead, 1 cun long from Shenting（DU₂₄）straight downward along the meridian.

A. 1. 2 MS₂ Epangxian I（额旁1线）

Line 1 lateral to forehead, 1 cun long from Meichong（BL₃）straight downward along the meridian.

A. 1. 3 MS₃ Epangxian II（额旁2线）

Line 2 lateral to forehead, 1 cun long from Toulinqi（GB₁₅）straight downward along the meridian.

A. 1. 4 MS₄ Epangxian III（额旁3线）

Line 3 lateral to forehead, 1 cun long from the point 0.75 cun medial to Touwei（ST₈）straight downward.

A. 1. 5 MS₅ Dingzhongxian（顶中线）

Middle line of vertex, from Baihui（DU₂₀）to Qianding（DU₂₁）along the midline of head.

A. 1. 6 MS₆ Dingnie Qianxiexian（顶颞前斜线）

Anterior oblique line of vertex – temporal, from Qian Sishencong（EX – HN₁）oblique to Xuanli（GB₆）.

A. 1. 7 MS₇ Dingnie Houxiexian（顶颞后斜线）

Posterior oblique line of vertex – temporal, from Baihui（DU₂₀）obliquely to Qubin（GB₇）.

A. 1. 8 MS₈ Dingpangxian I（顶旁1线）

Line 1 lateral to vertex, 1.5 cun long lateral to middle line of vertex, 1.5 cun long from Chenguang（BL₆）backward along the meridian.

A. 1. 9 MS₉ Dingpangxian II（顶旁2线）

Line 2 lateral to vertex, 2.25 cun lateral to middle line of vertex, 1.5 cun long from Zhengying（GB₁₇）backward along the meridian.

A. 1. 10 MS₁₀ Nieqianxian（颞前线）

Anterior temporal line, from Hanyan（GB₄）to Xuanli（GB₆）.

A. 1. 11 MS₁₁ Niehouxian（颞后线）

Posterior temporal line, from Shuaigu（GB₈）to Qubin（GB₇）.

A. 1. 12 MS₁₂ Zhenshang Zhengzhongxian（枕上正中线）

Upper – middle line of occiput, from Qianjian（DU₁₈）to Naohui（DU₁₇）.

A. 1. 13 MS₁₃ Zhenshang Pangxian（枕上旁线）

Upper – middle line of occiput, 0.5 cun lateral and parallel to upper – middle line of occiput.

A. 1. 14 MS₁₄ Zhenxia Pangxian（枕下旁线）

Lower – lateral line of occiput, 2 cun long from Yuzhen（BL₉）straight downward.

A.2　定位与主治
A.2.1　额区（图A1）

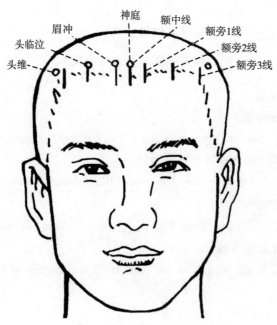

图A1　头正面头针穴线图示

A.2.1.1　额中线

定位：在额部正中，前发际上下各0.5寸，即神庭穴（DU$_{24}$）向下针1寸，属督脉。

主治：头痛、强笑、自哭、失眠、健忘、多梦、癫、狂、痫、鼻病等。

A.2.1.2　额旁1线

定位：在额部，额中线外侧直对目内眦角，发际上下各0.5寸，即眉冲穴（BL$_3$）沿经向下刺1寸，属足太阳膀胱经。

主治：冠心病、心绞痛、支气管哮喘、支气管炎、失眠等上焦病证。

A.2.1.3　额旁2线

定位：在额部，额旁1线的外侧，直对瞳孔，发际上下各0.5寸，即头临泣（GB$_{15}$）向下针1寸，属足少阳胆经。

主治：急慢性胃炎、胃十二指肠溃疡、肝胆疾病等中焦病证。

A.2.1.4　额旁3线

定位：在额部，额旁2线的外侧，自头维穴（ST$_8$）的内侧0.75寸处，发际上下各0.5寸，共1寸，属足少阳胆经与足阳明胃经之间。

主治：功能性子宫出血、阳痿、遗精、子宫脱垂、尿频、尿急等下焦病证。

A.2.2 顶区（图 A2～A3）

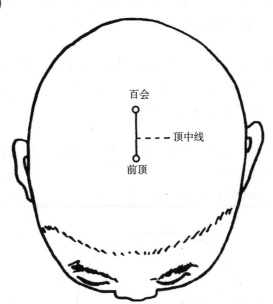

图 A2　头顶头针穴线图示

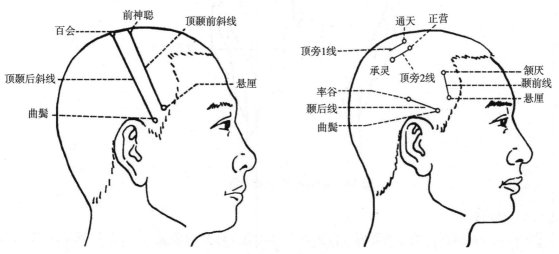

图 A3　头侧面头针穴线图示

A.2.2.1 顶中线

定位：在头顶正中线上，自百会穴（DU$_{20}$）向前 1.5 寸至前顶穴（DU$_{21}$），属督脉。

主治：腰、腿、足病证（如瘫痪、麻木、疼痛）、皮层性多尿、小儿夜尿、脱肛、胃下垂、子宫脱垂、高血压、头顶痛等。

A.2.2.2 顶颞前斜线

定位：在头部侧面，自前神聪穴至悬厘穴（GB$_6$）的连线，此线斜穿足太阳膀胱经、足少阳胆经。

主治：对侧肢体中枢性运动功能障碍。将全线分成 5 等分，上 1/5 治疗对侧下肢中枢性瘫痪；中 2/5 治疗对侧上肢中枢性瘫痪；下 2/5 治疗对侧中枢性面瘫、运动性失语、流涎、脑动脉硬化等。

A.2.2.3 顶颞后斜线

定位：在头部侧面，自百会穴（DU$_{20}$）至曲鬓穴（GB$_7$）的连线。此线斜穿督脉、足太阳膀胱经和足少阳胆经。

主治：对侧肢体中枢性感觉障碍。将全线分成 5 等分，上 1/5 治疗对侧下肢感觉异常；中 2/5 治疗对侧上肢感觉异常；下 2/5 治疗对侧头面部感觉异常。

A.2.2.4　顶旁 1 线

定位：在头顶部，顶中线左右各旁开 1.5 寸的两条平行线，自承光穴（BL_6）起向后针 1.5 寸，属足太阳膀胱经。

主治：腰、腿、足病证，如瘫痪、麻木、疼痛等。

A.2.2.5　顶旁 2 线

定位：在头顶部，顶旁 1 线的外侧，两线相距 0.75 寸，距正中线 2.25 寸，自正营穴（GB_{17}）起沿经线向后针 1.5 寸，属足少阳胆经。

主治：肩、臂、手病证，如瘫痪、麻木、疼痛等。

A.2.3　颞区（图 A4）

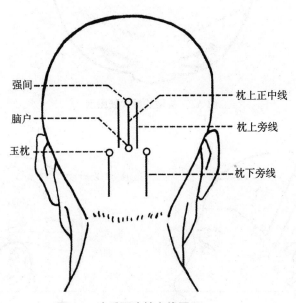

图 A4　头后面头针穴线图示

A.2.3.1　颞前线

定位：在头部侧面，颞部两鬓内，自额角下部向前发际处的颔厌穴（GB_4）到悬厘穴（GB_7），属足少阳胆经。

主治：偏头痛、运动性失语、周围性面神经麻痹及口腔疾病等。

A.2.3.2　颞后线

定位：在头部侧面，颞部耳上方，耳尖直上自率谷穴（GB_8）到曲鬓穴（GB_7），属足少阳胆经。

主治：偏头痛、眩晕、耳聋、耳鸣等。

A.2.4　枕区

A.2.4.1　枕上正中线

定位：在枕部，枕外粗隆上方正中的垂直线，自强间穴（DU_{18}）至脑户穴（DU_{17}），属督脉。

主治：眼病。

A.2.4.2　枕上旁线

定位：在枕部，枕上正中线平行向外 0.5 寸。

主治：皮层性视力障碍、白内障、近视眼、目赤肿痛等眼病。

A.2.4.3 枕下旁线

定位：在枕部，从膀胱经玉枕穴（BL$_9$）向下引一直线，长2寸，属足太阳膀胱经。

主治：小脑疾病引起的平衡障碍、后头痛、腰背两侧痛。

附 录 B

（规范性附录）

头针异常情况的处理和预防

B.1 晕针

B.1.1 临床表现

在头针操作过程中，患者突然出现精神疲倦，头晕目眩，面色苍白，恶心欲吐，多汗，心慌，四肢发冷，血压下降，脉象沉细，或神志昏迷，扑倒在地，唇甲青紫，二便失禁，脉微细欲绝。

B.1.2 处理方法

应立即停止针刺，将针全部起出，使患者平卧，注意保暖。轻者仰卧片刻，给饮温开水或糖水，即可恢复。重者在上述处理的基础上，可刺水沟、内关、足三里，灸百会、关元、气海等穴，即可恢复。若仍不省人事，呼吸微弱，可考虑配合其他治疗，采用急救措施。

B.1.3 预防措施

B.1.3.1 对初诊患者要详细询问是否做过针刺治疗，有无晕针史，仔细审察体质强弱，预先做好有关治疗的解释工作。对不愿进行头针治疗者，决不能勉强。

B.1.3.2 有晕针史者，应选择舒适持久的体位，最好采用卧位，选穴宜少，一般不做强刺激手法，可沿皮浅刺而不留针，即便必须用强刺激手法，其频率、幅度、用力程度宜适当，要在患者能耐受的情况下，逐步使其有一个适应过程。

B.1.3.3 饥饿、劳累、过饱、醉酒时，不应采用头针治疗。

B.1.3.4 医者在针刺治疗过程中，要精神集中，随时注意观察患者的神色，询问患者的感觉，一旦有不适等晕针先兆，可及早采取处理措施，防患于未然。

B.2 滞针

B.2.1 临床表现

滞针在头针治疗中常易发生。针刺入头皮以后，医者感觉针下涩滞，捻转、提插、出针均感困难，患者则感觉痛剧。

B.2.2 处理方法

发生滞针后，应适当延长留针时间，嘱患者身心放松，并在针体周围轻柔按摩。

B.2.3 预防措施

滞针主要发生于单向快速捻转的情况下。临床上，要注意手法用力均匀和适当，避免用蛮力，避免单向捻转。

B.3 弯针和断针

B.3.1 临床表现

针体在头穴内、外发生弯曲或折断。

B.3.2 处理方法

出现弯针和断针后，不能再行提插、捻转等手法。如针柄轻微弯曲，应慢慢将针起出；若弯曲角度过大时，应顺着弯曲方向将针起出。切忌强行拔针，以免将针体折断而留在体内。如果已经发生断针，若尚有残端显露于体表外，可用手或镊子将针起出。若断端与皮肤相平或稍凹陷于体内者，可用左手拇、食二指垂直向下挤压针孔两旁，使断针暴露体外，右手持镊子将针取出。若断针完全深入皮下，应在 X 线下定位，手术取出。

B.3.3 预防措施

应认真检查针具质量，凡有折痕、锈蚀的毫针绝不能使用。另外，在留针和行针过程中，应嘱咐患者避免针柄被外力碰触，以防发生弯针和断针。

B.4 血肿

B.4.1 临床表现

由于头皮部血管丰富，常易发生进针、留针时局部疼痛和出针后皮下出血而引起的肿痛，称为血肿。

B.4.2 处理方法

若微量的皮下出血而局部小块青紫时，一般不必处理，可以自行消退。若局部肿胀疼痛较剧，青紫面积大，应先做冷敷止血，再做热敷，或在局部轻轻揉按，以促使局部瘀血消散吸收。

B.4.3 预防措施

仔细检查针具，熟悉人体头部的解剖学位置关系，避开血管针刺，出针时立即用消毒干棉球揉按压迫针孔。对于容易出血的患者，出针宜轻快，并马上按压针孔，留针或不留针。